My First Time
Going to the De

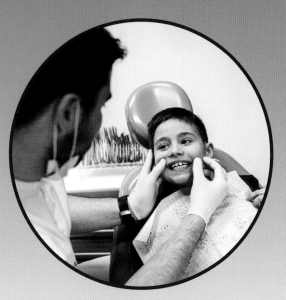

by Jeri Cipriano

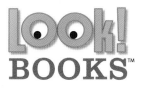
BOOKS™

Red Chair Press   Egremont, Massachusetts

Look! Books are produced and published by Red Chair Press:

Red Chair Press LLC   PO Box 333   South Egremont, MA 01258-0333

FREE Educator Guides at www.redchairpress.com/free-resources

Publisher's Cataloging-In-Publication Data

Names: Cipriano, Jeri, author.

Title: Going to the dentist / by Jeri Cipriano.

Description: Egremont, Massachusetts : Red Chair Press, [2021] | Series:
    Look! books. My first time | Includes index and a list of resources for
    further reading. | Interest age level: 005-008. | Summary: "Healthy
    teeth are important, and a trip to the dentist helps keep them shiny
    and strong. Get an inside look at the people who work hard to keep your
    teeth looking and feeling their best. Discover what happens during a
    dental exam and learn about the tools used to clean your teeth"--
    Provided by publisher.

Identifiers: ISBN 9781643710969 (RLB hardcover) | ISBN 9781643711027
    (softcover) | ISBN 9781643711089 (ebook)

Subjects: LCSH: Dentists--Juvenile literature. | Dental care--Utilization--
    Juvenile literature. | Teeth--Care and hygiene--Juvenile literature. |
    CYAC: Dentists. | Dental care. | Teeth--Care and hygiene.

Classification: LCC RK63 .C56 2021 (print) | LCC RK63 (ebook) | DDC
    617.6/0232--dc23

LCCN: 2020948763

Photo credits: iStock

Printed in United States of America
0122 2P   CGF21

Table of Contents

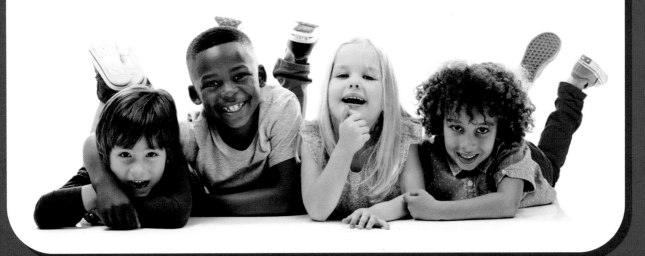

Your Teeth

Your teeth are important. They help you bite and chew food. Teeth help you speak clearly. Teeth help you smile—and even whistle!

As a child, you have 20 "baby" teeth. These teeth begin to fall out when you are about 6 or 7 years old.

Good to Know

Two bottom teeth will be the first to go. Why? Because they were the first to come in. Teeth fall out in the same order they came in.

As You Grow

Right now, your **permanent** teeth are still growing. You can't see them. But they are there—inside your gums. If your tooth wiggles and feels loose, a permanent tooth is ready to push out and take its place.

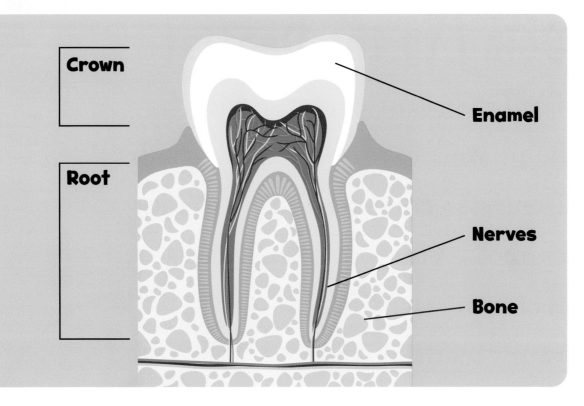

Crown

Root

Enamel

Nerves

Bone

Parts of a Tooth

The outside of a tooth—the part you see—is the **crown**. It is covered by **enamel**. This cover is harder than bone. Enamel protects the inside of your teeth. It covers the soft parts and the roots. Like trees, teeth have roots. Roots keep your teeth in place in your mouth.

Good to Know

Sometimes, you bite into something very cold or very hot. The *nerves* in your tooth let your brain know. Ouch!

Going to the Dentist

Dentists are doctors who help you care for your teeth. Dentists can see things you cannot. They use special tools to see inside your teeth.

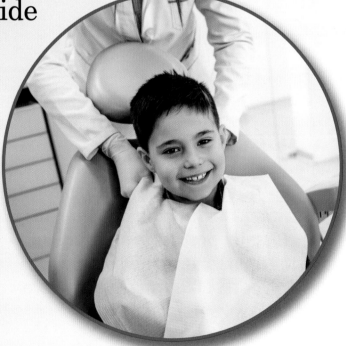

Going to the dentist about every six months helps keep your teeth healthy.

It's your turn to sit in the big dentist chair. This chair goes up and down. It tilts back so you can be comfortable. Open wide. The dentist shines a light in your mouth. First, the dentist counts your teeth.

Good to Know

A grown-up has 32 teeth in all.

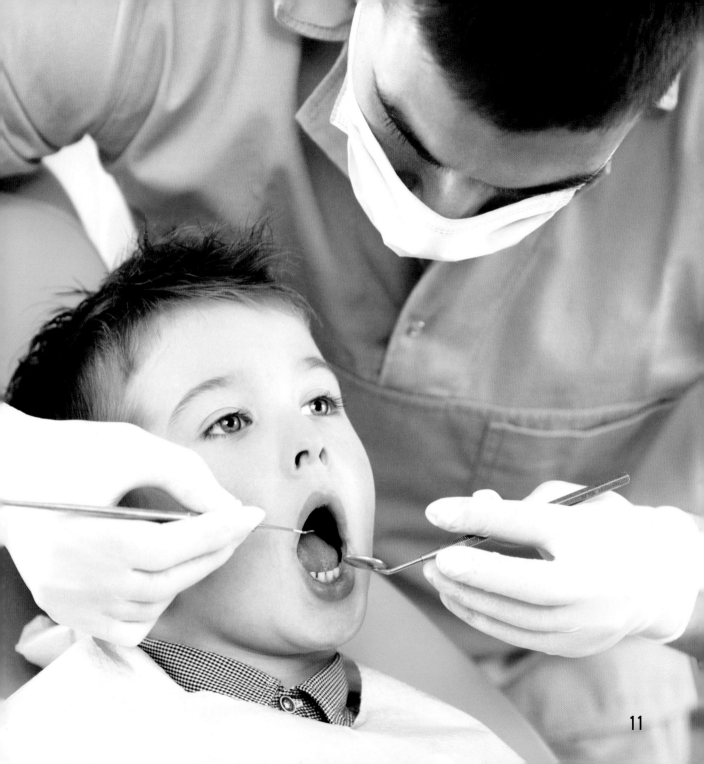

Dentist Tools

The dentist uses a small mirror to look at all parts of your mouth. The hooked, or curved, instrument is used to clean your teeth. Another tool polishes your teeth. It is soft but makes a funny buzzing sound.

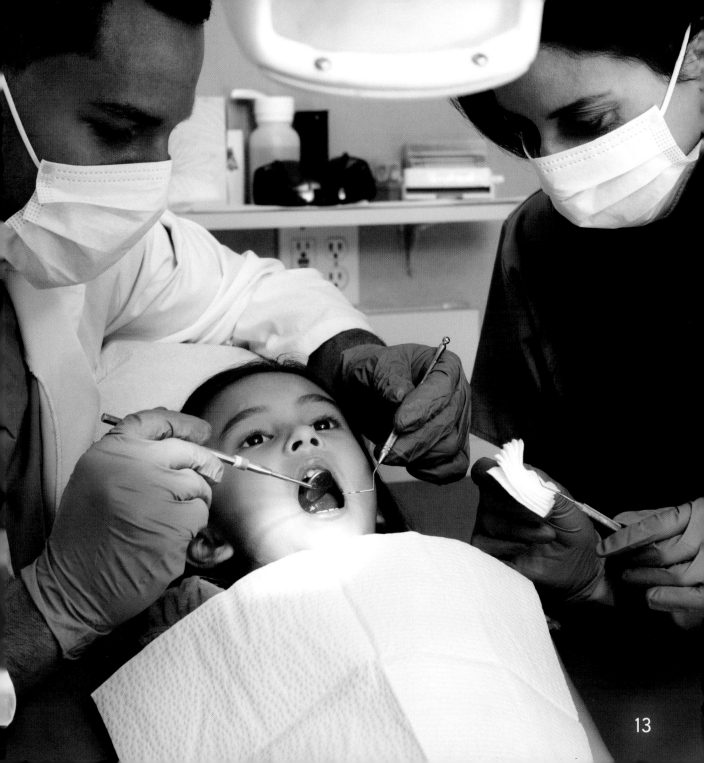

A Picture of Your Teeth

Before you leave, the dentist will want a picture of your teeth. The kind of picture a dentist looks at is an **X-ray**. The X-ray lets the dentist see inside, between, and around your teeth.

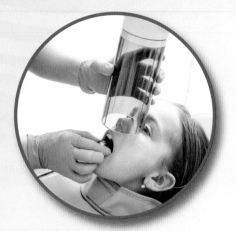

The dentist's helper puts a special camera against your cheek. The helper covers your throat and body with a heavy apron. Click. The picture is done.

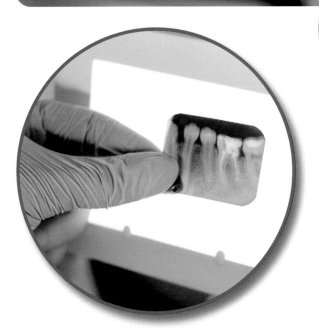

X-ray of a Tooth

This x-ray shows a **cavity**, or small hole in a tooth. The dentist will fill the hole to keep the tooth strong.

Taking Care of Your Teeth

How do you keep from getting cavities? One way is to brush your teeth twice each day—in the morning and at night.

Brush gently up, down, and around. Brush on each side. Open wide. Now brush the back of each tooth.

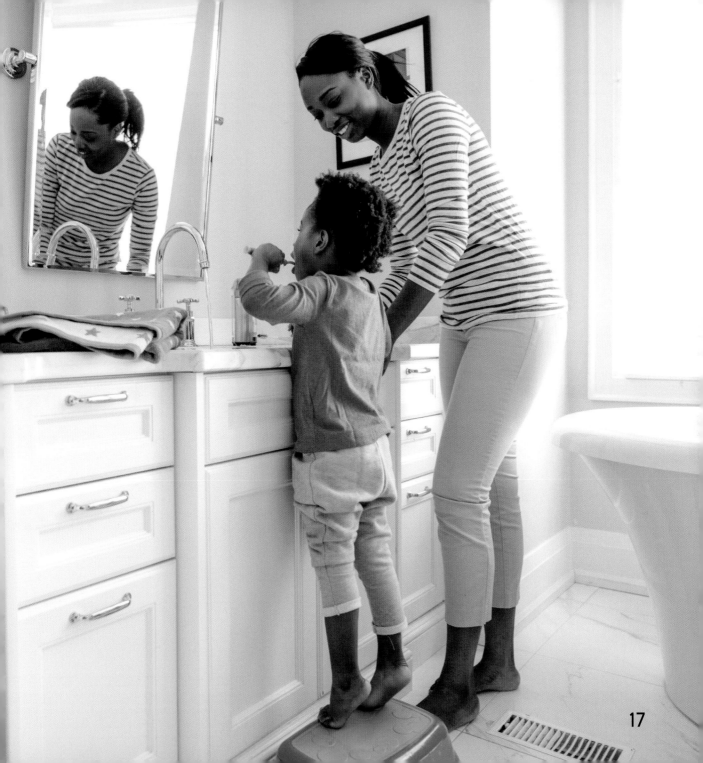

Experts say you should brush your teeth for two minutes. Press gently as you brush to sweep away food that is sticking to your teeth.

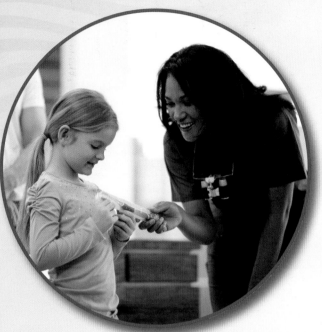

Good to Know

Replace your soft toothbrush with a new one every 3 to 4 months. Brush both the front and the back side of your teeth.

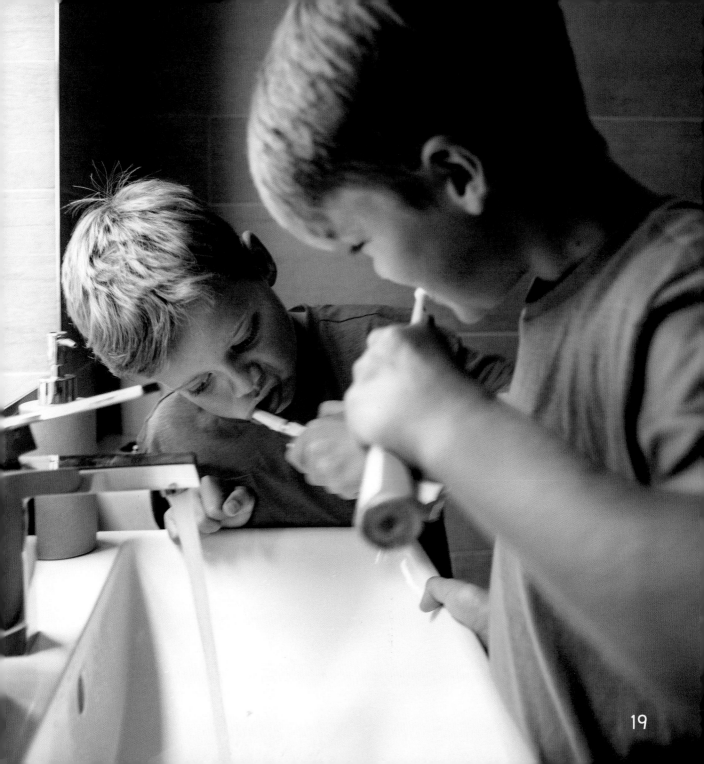

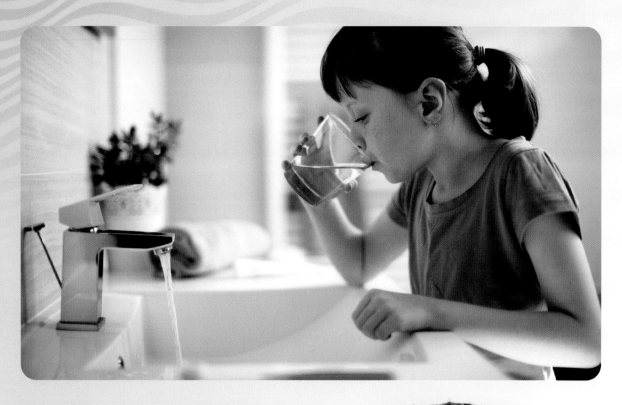

Eat Right and Floss

Foods that are too sweet, like candy and cake, make cavities. So, eat lots of fresh fruits and vegetables. Rinse your mouth with water after eating sticky foods.

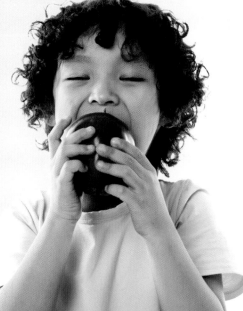

People use a small thread to clean between teeth. This is called dental floss. Sometimes floss comes with a little handle that makes it easy to use.

Time to Smile

What do you call bears without teeth?

Gummy bears.

Words to Keep

cavity: hole in a tooth caused by decay

expert: a person who knows something for sure

instrument: a device or tool

jawbone: upper and lower bones in mouth that hold the teeth

permanent: lasting for a very long time

Learn More at the Library

Check out these books to learn more.

Hoes, Bridget. *Let's Meet a Dentist.* Millbrook Press, 2013.

Schuh, Mari. *At the Dentist.* Capstone Press, 2008.

Smith, Penny. *A Trip to the Dentist.* DK Childrens' Books, 2006.

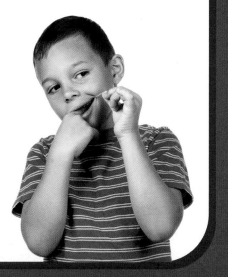

Index

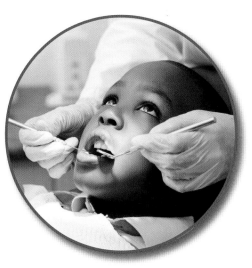

About the Author

Jeri Cipriano enjoys writing for children of all ages. She loves to learn new things she can share with others.

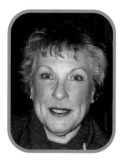